Mediterranean Diet

Instant Pot Cookbook with Delicious Recipes

LELA GIBSON

Copyright © 2018 Lela Gibson
All rights reserved.

CONTENTS

Introduction	6

Chapter 1: Mediterranean Instant Pot Breakfast Recipes — 8

French Crust less Meaty Quiche	8
French Omelet	10
Potato-Bacon Hash Browns	11
Breakfast Quinoa	13

Chapter 2: Mediterranean Instant Pot Soup Recipes — 14

Tortellini Soup with Sausage and Kale	14
Vegetarian Sausage and Gnocchi Soup	16
Moroccan Lentil Stew	18
Lebanese Chickpea Soup with Moghrabieh	20
Chicken & Smoked Sausage Stew	22
Butternut Squash Soup	24
Mediterranean Soup	26

Chapter 3: Mediterranean Instant Pot Main Course Recipes — 28

Chicken Parmesan Lasagna	28
Spaghetti Squash with Apple Juice	30
Mediterranean Collard Greens	32
Italian Red Pepper Chicken	34
Greek Stuffed Chicken Breasts	35

Shrimp Risotto	37
Italian Pulled Pork Ragu	39
Mediterranean Pork with Couscous	41
Instant Pot Lamb Curry	43
Vegetable Lasagna	45
Italian Eggplant and Lentils	47
Italian White Beans	49
Instant Pot Chicken	50
Chicken Shawarma	52
Mediterranean Beef	53
Rosemary Salmon	55
Lentil Risotto	56
Chapter 4: Mediterranean Instant Pot Dessert Recipes	**57**
Baked Apples	57
Peanut Butter Chocolate Cheesecake	58
Pots de Crème au Citron	60
Flan de Queso	62
Pears Stewed in Red Wine	64
I Need Your Help...	**66**
Preview of 'Air Fryer Cookbook'	**67**
Check Out My Other Books	**75**
Bonus: Subscribe To The Free Weight Loss Report	**79**

MEDITERRANEAN DIET

Introduction

I want to thank you and congratulate you for buying the book, 'Mediterranean Diet - Instant Pot Cookbook with Delicious Recipes.'

The Mediterranean cuisine is considered to be the best and tastiest cuisine in the world. Since it is based on traditional recipes and foods, it is quite popular among people who want to be healthy and fit without giving up on tasty food. It is an ancient cuisine that is a combination of a variety of equally rich cuisines including Greek, Levantine, Provençal (French), Ottoman (Turkish), Maghreb, Italian, Spanish and Portuguese.

The Mediterranean diet focuses on consuming products that are primarily plant-based for instance fruits and vegetables, legumes, whole grains and nuts. Butter is replaced with olive oil or canola oil and there is an extra focus on the use of fresh and dried herbs to make the food tastier. A variety of vegetables, fruit and meats are used in this cuisine, which makes it wholesome, healthy, tasty and satiating.

In this book, you will find delicious and mouth-watering Mediterranean diet recipes that can be cooked in an instant pot. Most of the recipes are quick and easy to make, making it popular among amateur cooks as well. They are modified slightly to suit the concept of healthy eating; thus, are combine healthy foods that are fresh, as well as producing tasty meals.

The recipes mentioned here try to incorporate the best characteristics of the cuisine in a modern, health-based diet. All the recipes are tried, tested and tasted. You can trust them blindfolded on giving a healthy and tasty outcome. Let your inner glutton come out and get in the kitchen right away!

Thanks again for buying this book, I hope you enjoy it!

Chapter 1: Mediterranean Instant Pot Breakfast Recipes

French Crust less Meaty Quiche

Serves: 8

Cook time: 20 minutes

Ingredients:

- 12 large eggs, whisked
- Salt to taste
- 2 cups ground sausage, cooked
- 8 slices bacon, cooked, crumbled
- 1 cup ham, diced
- 4 large green onions, chopped
- 1 cup milk
- 2 cups cheese, shredded
- Pepper to taste

Method:

1. Add eggs, milk, salt and pepper into a bowl and whisk well.

2. Add meat, cheese, and green onions into a greased soufflé dish.

3. Pour egg mixture over it and stir. Cover loosely with aluminum foil.

4. Pour 1 ½ cups water into the instant pot. Place a trivet in it.

5. Place the soufflé dish on the trivet.

6. Close the lid. Select 'Manual' button and timer for 20 minutes. Let the pressure release naturally.

7. Remove the dish. Sprinkle some extra cheese on top if desired and broil for a few minutes.

8. Slice and serve.

French Omelet

Serves: 2

Cook time: 5 minutes

Ingredients:

- 4 eggs, separated
- Salt to taste
- Pepper to taste
- 4 tablespoons water
- 1/3 cup ham, finely chopped
- 1/3 cup cheese, shredded
- Cooking spray

Method:

1. Whisk whites until fluffy. Add yolks and whisk again.
2. Spray the inner pot with cooking spray. Pour eggs into the pot.
3. Sprinkle ham, cheese, salt and pepper over it.
4. Select 'Steam' button and timer for 5 minutes.
5. When done, carefully remove on to a plate.
6. Cut into 2 equal parts and serve.

Potato-Bacon Hash Browns

Serves: 4

Cook time: 15 minutes

Ingredients:

- Pepper, freshly ground
- Salt
- 2 tablespoons parsley, chopped
- 225 grams crumbled bacon
- 1 kg sweet potatoes, washed and peeled
- 2 tablespoons olive oil

Method:

1. Process the sweet potatoes in a food processor or grate them. Using a strainer, rinse and let it sit under running water for 30 seconds.
2. Using paper towels, thoroughly dry the potatoes as this helps get crispier hash.
3. Add oil into an Instant Pot and press the sauté button. Once the oil is hot, add in the potatoes, season with salt and pepper then sauté for 5-6 minutes until brown.

4. Add in parsley and bacon. Mix well and then press the bacon and potato down firmly using a wide spatula.

5. Lock the lid and cook for 6-7 minutes at manual low pressure. Quick release pressure.

6. Serve hot with some fruit juice.

Breakfast Quinoa

Serves: 6

Cook Time: 10 to 15 minutes

Ingredients

- Pinch of salt
- 1/4 teaspoon cinnamon, ground
- 1/2 teaspoon vanilla
- 2 tablespoons maple syrup
- 2 1/4 cups water
- 1 1/2 cups quinoa, uncooked and well rinsed

Directions

1. Add in cinnamon, vanilla, maple syrup, water, quinoa and salt into the cooking pot of your instant pot,
2. Cook for 1 minute at high pressure.
3. Release the pressure and open the lid after the valve drops.
4. Fluff the quinoa and then serve it hot with slice almonds, berries and milk.

Chapter 2: Mediterranean Instant Pot Soup Recipes

Tortellini Soup with Sausage and Kale

Serves: 4-5

Cook Time: 40 minutes

Ingredients:

- ½ pound ground sweet Italian sausage
- 1 stalk celery, chopped
- 1 carrot, chopped
- 1 medium onion, chopped
- 1 ½ cups lacinato kale, discard hard ribs and stems, chopped
- 2 cloves garlic, minced
- Freshly ground black pepper to taste
- Salt to taste
- 3 tablespoons dry white wine or sherry
- 7.5 ounces canned, diced tomatoes
- 4 cups chicken stock
- ½ pound fresh 3 cheese tortellini
- ½ teaspoon dried oregano

- ½ teaspoon dried basil
- ½ teaspoon dried parsley
- Parmesan cheese, grated to garnish

Method:

1. Select 'Sauté' button. Add sausage and cook until brown. Break it simultaneously as it cooks.

2. Add celery and onion and sauté for 3-4 minutes. Add garlic and sauté for a few seconds until fragrant.

3. Add salt, pepper and sherry. Scrape the bottom of the pot to remove any browned bits that are stuck.

4. Add rest of the ingredients and stir.

5. Close the slid. Select 'Soup' button. When the timer goes off, quick release excess pressure.

6. Add tortellini and kale. Select 'Slow cook' button and set the timer for 30 minutes.

7. Ladle into soup bowls. Garnish with Parmesan cheese and serve.

Vegetarian Sausage and Gnocchi Soup

Serves: 3

Cook Time: 4 hours

Ingredients:

- 3 vegetarian sausages, sliced
- 5 ounces gnocchi
- 1 carrot, peeled, chopped
- 1 small onion, chopped
- 1 celery rib, chopped
- 2 cups spinach, chopped
- 1 cup mushrooms, sliced
- 10 ounces canned diced tomatoes with Italian seasoning
- 2 cups vegetable broth
- Freshly ground black pepper to taste
- Salt to taste
- ½ teaspoon Italian seasoning or to taste

To serve:

- Handful fresh parsley, chopped
- Parmesan cheese, grated, as required

Method:

1. Add all the ingredients except spinach and gnocchi into the instant pot.
2. Close the lid. Select 'Slow cook' button and set the timer for 3 hours.
3. Add gnocchi and spinach during the last 50-60 minutes of cooking.
4. Ladle into soup bowls. Garnish with Parmesan cheese and parsley and serve.

Moroccan Lentil Stew

Serves: 3

Ingredients:

- 1 stalk celery, chopped
- 1 carrot, chopped
- 1 medium onion, chopped
- 2 cups kale, discard hard ribs and stems, chopped
- 1 ½ cups cauliflower, chopped
- 2 cloves garlic, minced
- Freshly ground black pepper to taste
- Salt to taste
- 1 teaspoon paprika
- ½ teaspoon turmeric powder
- ½ teaspoon ground cumin
- ½ teaspoon ground coriander
- 1 teaspoon olive oil
- ¾ cup dried red lentils, rinsed
- 1 tablespoon tomato paste
- 10 ounces canned diced tomatoes

- 3 cups vegetable broth
- 1 tablespoon lemon juice
- ¼ cup fresh cilantro

Method:

1. Add all the ingredients except lemon juice and cilantro into the instant pot and stir.

2. Close the lid. Select 'Meat /Stew' button. Let the pressure release naturally.

3. Add lemon juice and cilantro and stir.

4. Ladle into bowls and serve.

Lebanese Chickpea Soup with Moghrabieh

Serves: 3

Ingredients:

- 1 medium onion, chopped
- 1 carrot, diced
- 1 rib celery, diced
- 2 cloves garlic, minced
- ¼ teaspoon paprika
- ½ teaspoon ground cumin
- 1/8 teaspoon ground allspice
- A pinch saffron, lightly crushed
- 2 inch stick cinnamon
- 1/8 teaspoon chili powder or cayenne pepper
- 1/8 teaspoon ground ginger
- 1 bay leaf
- 1 ½ cups cooked chickpeas
- 2 tablespoons Moghrabieh (Lebanese couscous)
- ¼ cup fresh parsley, chopped
- Salt to taste

- 1 tablespoon lemon juice
- 4-5 cups vegetable broth
- Cooking spray

Method:

1. Spray the inside of the instant pot with cooking spray. Select 'Sauté' button.

2. When the pot is heated, add carrot, onion and celery and sauté until the onions are light brown.

3. Add garlic and sauté until fragrant. Add paprika, cumin, allspice, saffron, cinnamon, chili powder, ginger and bay leaf. Sauté for a minute.

4. Add chickpeas and stir for a couple of minutes.

5. Add stock and moghrabieh.

6. Close the lid. Select 'Porridge' button. When the timer goes off, let the pressure release naturally for 5 minutes after which release excess pressure.

Chicken & Smoked Sausage Stew

Serves: 6

Cook Time : 15 to 20 minutes

Ingredients:

- 1 bay leaf
- 1/4 teaspoon cayenne
- 1/4 teaspoon black pepper
- 1/2 teaspoon red chili flakes, crushed
- 1/2 teaspoon smoked paprika
- 1 teaspoon thyme
- 1 teaspoon salt
- 6 cloves garlic
- 1/4 cup parsley
- 2 cups bone broth or water
- 2 large carrots
- 3 bell peppers
- 2 stalks celery

- 1 medium white onion

- 6 cups tomatoes, chopped

- 1 tablespoon coconut oil

- 1 pound andouille pork sausage

- 1 pound boneless, skinless chicken thighs

- Hot sauce, optional:

Method:

1. Into the Instant Pot, heat coconut oil on sauté setting. Then add in sausage and chicken to the pan until cooked through.

2. Meanwhile, slice the onions, chop the celery and carrots and dice the bell peppers. Now remove the meat from the pressure cooker and set it aside.

3. Sauté the veggies as you stir regularly. Then mince garlic and add into the cooking veggies. Follow with chopped tomatoes and broth. Allow the mixture to simmer on sauté setting.

4. Once the sausage and chicken have cooled down, slice into bite-size chunks and return to the pot. Add the spices.

5. Mince the parsley, add it into the meat mixture and stir. Lock the lid in place and set the Instant Pot to Soup option, and cook for about 5 10 minutes.

Once ready, serve the chicken with hot sauce.

Butternut Squash Soup

Serves: 4

Cook Time: 10-15 minutes

Ingredients:

- 1 teaspoon dried tarragon
- ½ teaspoon nutmeg, ground
- 1 teaspoon cinnamon
- ½ teaspoon turmeric
- 1 ½ teaspoons curry powder
- 1 teaspoon Himalayan pink salt
- 2 tablespoons coconut oil
- 2 cloves garlic - crushed
- 1 inch ginger -peeled
- 1 small-medium onion - cubed
- 3 cups bone broth or chicken broth
- 2 cups of sweet potatoes, cubed
- 2 cups of butternut squash, cubed
- 1 teaspoon walnuts, chopped
- 1 teaspoon fresh parsley

Mediterranean Soup

Serves: 4

Cook Time: 30 minutes

Ingredients:

2 large sprigs of thyme, fresh

2 bay leaves

1 teaspoon salt

6 cups pork stock

1 tablespoon balsamic vinegar

8 cups yellow onions

2 tablespoons coconut oil

Method:

1. Slice the onions into thin half-moons. Press Sauté button on Instant Pot and add in oil.

2. Cook the onions for about 15 minutes as you stir. Once they reduce and become transparent, add in balsamic vinegar.

3. Add in the stock, thyme, bay leaves and salt. Turn off the Instant Pot and close the lid ensuring it is set to "sealing" position.

Method:

1. Press the sauté button on your Instant Pot. Add in ginger, onions, coconut oil, garlic and salt and cook until the onions soften.

2. Add the rest of the ingredients apart from walnuts and parsley, and stir to incorporate. Close the lid and set the timer to 10 minutes.

3. Once cooked, release pressure naturally then carefully open the lid. You can then puree the mixture in the pot or process in a blender or food processor.

4. Garnish the soup with walnuts and parsley.

4. Set instant pot to high pressure and cook for 10 minutes. When cooked, natural release pressure and wait for all liquids to cool down.

5. Open the lid and discard thyme and bay leaves. With an immersion blender, puree to form soup.

Chapter 3: Mediterranean Instant Pot Main Course Recipes

Chicken Parmesan Lasagna

Serves: 5

Ingredients:

- 25 ounces marinara sauce
- 8 ounces low fat ricotta cheese
- 1 ½ cups chicken, boneless, skinless, cooked, chopped
- 4 ounces no boil lasagna noodles
- 1 ¼ cups part skim mozzarella cheese, shredded, divided

Method:

1. Spread about ½ cup marinara sauce on the bottom of the instant pot. Spread a single layer of lasagna noodles.
2. Next layer with ricotta cheese followed by ½ cup mozzarella cheese.
3. Next layer with half the chicken and ½ cup marinara sauce.
4. Spread another layer of lasagna noodles followed by the remaining chicken and ½ cup mozzarella cheese.

5. Spread the remaining noodles if any and the sauce.

6. Close the lid. Select 'Slow cook' button and set the timer for 2-3 hours.

7. Sprinkle remaining cheese on it during the last 10 minutes of cooking

Spaghetti Squash with Apple Juice

Serves: 4

Cook Time: 25 to 30 minutes

Ingredients:

2 tablespoons coconut oil

3/4 cup apple juice

1- 3 lbs spaghetti squash

Sea salt, to taste

Method:

1. Put the rack into the instant pot then pour in a cup of water into the Instant Pot.

2. Lock the lid in place, set the cooker to manual and time it for 20 minutes.

3. Once time elapses, quick release the pressure and open the lid. Remove the squash with hot pads and transfer to a cutting board.

4. Cut it in half and allow to cool. Then remove the rack and discard the water. Put the stainless steel insert into the cooking pot.

5. To prepare the sauce, pour apple juice into the insert and press sauté button. Simmer for 3 minutes until the liquid is reduced. At this point, add in coconut oil and once it melts, turn off the instant pot.

6. Scoop out the seeds from spaghetti squash and discard them. Scrape the squash noodles using a fork into a pot.

7. Finally season with sea salt, and toss to coat. Adjust seasonings and serve.

Mediterranean Collard Greens

Serves: 2

Cook Time : 20 to 30 minutes

Ingredients:

- 1 small onion, sliced thin
- 1 bunch fresh collard greens
- 1/2 teaspoon salt
- 1 tablespoon balsamic vinegar
- 3 minced garlic cloves
- 2 tablespoons diced tomatoes
- 2 tablespoons olive oil
- 1/2 cup chicken broth

Method:

1. Begin by soaking the collard greens to remove dirt for around 30 minutes.

2. In an Instant Pot, mix together tomato puree, garlic, chicken broth, vinegar, oil and onion and stir thoroughly.

3. Meanwhile, remove the greens from the sink one by one while not disturbing the water to ensure the dirt settles at the bottom of the sink.

4. Cut the thick stems at the base of the greens, chopping them into tiny pieces, before placing them on each other.

5. Now roll them to form cigar-shaped bundles and then cut the greens into 1-2 inches pieces.

6. Toss the greens with salt, and then add them into the instant pot.

7. Add the collard greens into the instant pot and toss to coat with the oil mixture, and then cook on sauté setting for 20 minutes. When done, quick release the pressure and carefully open the lid. Serve.

Italian Red Pepper Chicken

Serves: 3

Ingredients:

- 1 pound chicken breast, skinless, boneless, chopped
- 2 medium red peppers, sliced
- 1 large clove garlic, minced
- 1 medium onion, sliced
- 10 ounces canned, diced, fire roasted tomatoes
- 1 tablespoon balsamic vinegar
- ½ teaspoon red pepper flakes or to taste
- ½ teaspoon salt
- ½ teaspoon pepper
- 2 teaspoons Italian seasoning

Method:

1. Add all the ingredients into the instant pot. Mix well.
2. Close the lid. Select 'Poultry' button. When the poultry cycle completes, let the pressure release naturally.

Greek Stuffed Chicken Breasts

Serves: 3

Ingredients:

- 3 chicken breasts (6 ounces each)
- ¼ cup roasted red peppers, chopped
- ½ cup canned artichoke hearts, chopped
- 1 ½ cups spinach, finely chopped
- 2 tablespoons black olives, sliced
- 2 ounces low fat feta cheese
- ½ teaspoon garlic powder
- ½ teaspoon dried oregano
- Salt to taste
- Pepper to taste
- ¾ cup chicken broth

Method:

1. Add spinach, red pepper, spinach, oregano, feta and garlic into a bowl. Mix well.
2. Sprinkle salt and pepper over the chicken.

3. Take a sharp knife and make a slit in the center of each chicken breast so that a pocket is created.

4. Stuff the spinach mixture into the pockets. Place chicken in the instant pot with the stuffed part facing up. Pour broth all around the chicken.

5. Close the lid. Select 'Slow cook' button and timer for 2 hours or until cooked.

Shrimp Risotto

Serves: 6-8

Ingredients:

- 6 tablespoons olive oil
- 2 shallots, minced
- 4 cups Arborio rice, rinsed
- 8 tablespoons butter, unsalted
- 6 medium cloves garlic minced
- 1 ½ cups cooking sake
- 5 tablespoons miso paste
- 4 teaspoons Japanese soy sauce
- 8 cups fish stock, unsalted
- ¼ teaspoon baking soda
- 1 pound tiger prawns or shrimp, frozen, unpeeled, thawed
- 1 teaspoon kosher salt
- 4 green onions, thinly sliced
- ¼ cup parmesan cheese, finely grated + extra to garnish
- Salt to taste
- Pepper to taste

Method:

1. To dry brine the shrimp (optional): Pat the shrimp dry with paper towels. Add into a bowl. Add baking soda and kosher salt and mix well. Refrigerate for 30 minutes.

2. Select 'Sauté' button and press 'Adjust' button once. Heat the pot until the indicator shows 'Hot'.

3. Add oil and butter. When the butter melts, add shallots and garlic and sauté until translucent.

4. Add shrimp and cook for 1 minute on each side. Remove the shrimp with a slotted spoon and set aside. Let the butter – oil mixture remain in the pot.

5. Add rice and sauté until the rice turns opaque. Add soy sauce and miso and mix well.

6. Add cooking sake. Scrape the bottom of the pot with a wooden spoon. Let it cook for a couple of minutes.

7. Close the lid. Select 'Rice' button. When the timer goes off, add green onions and cheese and stir.

8. Add salt and pepper and stir.

9. Meanwhile, peel the shrimp.

10. Divide the risotto among serving plates. Divide the shrimp among the plates. Sprinkle Parmesan cheese on top and serve.

Italian Pulled Pork Ragu

Serves: 5

Ingredients:

- 9 ounces pork tenderloin
- 3 cloves garlic, peeled, smashed
- 3.5 ounces jarred roasted red peppers
- 1 large red onion, chopped
- 1 can (14.5 ounces) crushed tomatoes
- 1 tablespoon fresh oregano, chopped
- 1 sprig fresh thyme
- 2 teaspoons fresh parsley, chopped, divided
- 1 bay leaf
- Pepper to taste
- ½ teaspoon kosher salt
- 1 teaspoon oil

Method:

1. Select 'Sauté' button. Add oil and heat.

2. Sprinkle salt and pepper over the pork and cook until light brown.

3. Add rest of the ingredients except 1-teaspoon parsley and stir. Press 'Cancel'

4. Close the lid. Select 'Meat / Stew' button. When the timer goes off, let the pressure release naturally.

5. Remove the meat with a slotted spoon and place on your work area.

6. When cool enough to handle, shred with a pair of forks.

7. Add it back into the pot. Heat thoroughly using the 'Sauté' button. Transfer into a bowl. Garnish with parsley.

8. Serve over pasta.

Mediterranean Pork with Couscous

Serves: 2

Ingredients:

- 1-1 ½ pounds pork loin, boneless, trimmed of fat
- ½ cup chicken broth
- 1 teaspoon garlic powder
- 1/8 teaspoon dried rosemary
- 1/8 teaspoon dried thyme
- 1/8 teaspoon dried marjoram
- 1 teaspoon dried sage
- ½ teaspoon dried basil
- ½ teaspoon dried oregano
- 1 teaspoon paprika
- 1 cup couscous, cook according to the instructions on the package
- 1 tablespoon olive oil

Method:

1. Add oil, broth, herbs and spices into a bowl. Mix well.
2. Take a paring knife and make small cuts in the pork roast.
3. Place the roast in the instant pot. Pour the spice mixture over the pork.
4. Close the lid. Select 'Slow cook' button and timer for 3-4 hours or until the pork is done.
5. Remove the meat with a slotted spoon and place on your work area.
6. When cool enough to handle, shred with a pair of forks.
7. Add it back into the pot. Heat thoroughly using the 'Sauté' button. Transfer into a bowl.
8. Serve pork with the gravy over couscous.

Instant Pot Lamb Curry

Serves: 3

Ingredients:

- ¾ pound lamb stew meat, cubed
- ½ inch fresh ginger, grated
- 1 tablespoon lime juice
- Pepper to taste
- Salt to taste
- ½ tablespoon ghee
- 1 teaspoon garam masala or yellow curry powder
- 2 cloves garlic, minced
- ½ teaspoon turmeric powder- to be used only if using garam masala
- ¼ cup coconut milk or more if required
- 7 ounces canned diced tomatoes
- 1 small onion, chopped
- 1 small zucchini, diced
- 1 large carrot, sliced
- Handful fresh cilantro, chopped

Method:

1. Add garlic, ginger, meat, coconut milk, lime juice, pepper and salt into a bowl. Mix well. Cover and refrigerator for 2-8 hours.

2. Remove from the refrigerator and add into the instant pot.

3. Also add tomatoes with its juice, ghee, carrots, onion and garam masala. Mix well.

4. Close the lid. Select 'Manual' and set the temperature for 20 minutes. When the timer goes off, let the pressure release naturally for 15 minutes after which release the remaining pressure.

5. Select 'Sauté' button and press 'Adjust' button twice. Add zucchini and stir. Let it simmer uncovered until the zucchini is soft and the soup thickened.

6. Garnish with cilantro and serve over rice or cauliflower rice.

Vegetable Lasagna

Serves: 4

Ingredients:

- 13-15 ounces Italian tomato sauce (marinara sauce)
- 5 thick lasagna noodles, broken
- ½ cup mushrooms, finely chopped
- ½ cup zucchini, finely chopped
- 2 cloves garlic, finely chopped
- 1 onion, finely chopped
- 1 small egg
- 7.5 ounces part skim ricotta cheese
- ½ cup mozzarella cheese, shredded
- 1 teaspoon dried basil or oregano
- 2 tablespoons fresh parsley

Method:

1. Spray the instant pot with cooking spray.
2. Mix together in a microwave safe bowl, mushroom, onion, garlic and zucchini.
3. Microwave on High for 2-4 minutes. Remove the vegetables and cool for a while. Squeeze excess moisture from the vegetables
4. Add ricotta, egg and basil in a bowl. Mix well.
5. Spread about 1/3 cup of tomato sauce at the bottom of the pot.
6. Lay about 1/3 of the lasagna pieces over it.
7. Make layers by spreading about 1/3 of each of the following; Vegetables, sauce, ricotta cheese mixture, mozzarella cheese and lasagna.
8. Repeat the above step twice.
9. Finally spread a thin layer of sauce.
10. Close the lid. Select 'Slow cook' button and set the timer for 3 hours.
11. When done, do not uncover, let it cool down for about an hour.
12. Sprinkle parsley over it. Slice and serve.

Italian Eggplant and Lentils

Serves: 3

Ingredients:

- 2 cups eggplant, cubed
- 1 medium onion, diced
- 2 cloves garlic, minced
- 3 tablespoons fresh basil, chopped
- ¾ cup dry lentils, rinsed
- ½ tablespoon olive oil
- 2 cloves garlic, minced
- 14 ounces canned crushed tomatoes
- ¾ cup vegetable broth
- ½ tablespoon dried Italian seasoning
- ¼ teaspoon red pepper flakes
- Salt to taste
- Pepper to taste

Method:

1. Sprinkle salt and pepper over the eggplant and place in the instant pot.

2. Add rest of the ingredients except basil.

3. Close the lid. Select 'Bean / Chili'. When the timer goes off, let the pressure release naturally for 5-6 minutes after which release excess pressure.

Italian White Beans

Serves: 3

Ingredients:

- 16-18 ounces canned diced tomatoes with Italian seasoning
- 4 cloves garlic, sliced
- 1 cup dry white beans, rinsed
- 3 tablespoons fresh parsley, chopped
- Pepper to taste
- Salt to taste
- 2 cups hot vegetable broth
- 2 teaspoons Italian seasoning
- 2 teaspoons balsamic vinegar

Method:

1. Add all the ingredients into the instant pot.
2. Close the lid. Close the lid. Select 'Bean / Chili'. When the timer goes off, let the pressure release naturally.

Instant Pot Chicken

Serves: 8

Cooking Time: 20 minutes

Ingredients

- ½ cup black olives
- 28oz can diced/chopped tomato
- Salt and black pepper to taste
- 2 teaspoons dried oregano
- 2 teaspoons dried parsley
- ½ teaspoon ground coriander seed
- ¼ teaspoon chili pepper
- 1 teaspoon onion powder
- 1 teaspoon smoked paprika
- 2 cups white onion, chopped
- 1 lb. organic chicken thighs (skinless and boneless)
- 2 tablespoons olive oil

Method:

1. Select the sauté function on your instant pot.

2. Add in olive oil into the pot and let it heat up. Once hot, add the chicken and sauté until brown; set aside

3. Add the onions and cook for around 5 minutes. Now add in the spices, seasonings, salt, pepper and diced tomatoes. Cook for around 2-3 minutes.

4. Return the chicken back into the instant pot and mix with all the ingredients until combined. Set to manual high pressure and cook for 8minutes.

5. Release the pressure, add in the olive and stir well. Serve this over vegetables, mashed potatoes, rice or pasta.

Chicken Shawarma

Serves: 4-6

Cook Time: 25 minutes

Ingredients:

- Kosher salt and freshly ground black pepper to taste
- 1/8 teaspoon ground cinnamon
- 1/4 teaspoon chili powder
- 1/4 teaspoon ground allspice
- 1/4 teaspoon granulated garlic
- 1/2 teaspoon turmeric
- 1 teaspoon paprika
- 1 teaspoon ground cumin
- 1 – 1.5 pounds boneless skinless chicken thighs
- 1 – 1.5 pounds boneless skinless chicken breasts

Method:

1. Slice the chicken into strips and put into your instant pot. Combine all the spices in a small bowl and pour this over the chicken, and then season with pepper and salt. Mix everything up so that the chicken is evenly coated with the spices.

2. Add the chicken broth and secure the lid. Select poultry setting and set the time for 15 minutes. Once time is up, release pressure and serve over sweet potatoes or veggies.

Mediterranean Beef

Serves: 6

Cook Time: 50 minutes

Ingredients

- 2 lb boneless beef chuck shoulder roast
- 1/2 cup chopped, pitted Medjool dates
- 1/4 cup good quality balsamic vinegar
- 1/4 cup red wine *if you don't have wine, just use more beef broth
- 1/2 cup beef broth
- 1 garlic clove, minced
- 2 tablespoons extra virgin olive oil
- 4 shallots, sliced
- 1 large onion, finely chopped
- 1/2 teaspoon dried oregano
- 1 teaspoon black pepper
- 1/2 teaspoon salt
- Parsley or fresh oregano for garnish

Method:

1. Mix salt, pepper and oregano and chop the meat into 2" pieces.

2. Place the meat in a plastic bag, add the spices, seal and shake for the spices to coat the meat.

3. Select the sauté function of your instant pot and add in the olive oil. Once the pot is hot, add the beef, garlic, shallots and onions. Sauté for around 4 minutes or until browned lightly making sure that you stir occasionally to prevent burning.

4. Add the vinegar, wine, broth and dates and stir to mix. Put the lid and lock to seal. To stop the sauté function, press cancel then select Manual and set timer for 40 minutes at high pressure.

5. Once ready, allow natural release and serve over brown rice, cauliflower rice or couscous.

Rosemary Salmon

Serves: 3

Cook Time: 15 minutes

Ingredients:

- 1 tablespoon olive oil
- 1/2 cup cherry tomatoes (halved)
- 1 sprig fresh rosemary
- 10 oz. fresh asparagus
- 1 lb. salmon (frozen, wild)
- salt and pepper (to taste after cooking)
- 1 tablespoon lemon juice (optional)

Method:

1. Pour a cup of water into your instant pot and put the wire rack. Put the salmon first, then the rosemary and then fresh asparagus. Select the manual button and adjust the time to 3 minutes.

2. Once ready, allow the pressure to release naturally, open the lid discard the rosemary sprig and serve. Add some tomatoes, drizzle some olive oil and season with some pepper and salt if desired. You can also drizzle some lemon juice.

Lentil Risotto

Serves: 4

Cook time: 15 minutes

Ingredients

- 1 cup dry lentils, soaked overnight
- 3¼ cups vegetable stock
- 2 garlic cloves, lightly mashed
- 1 cup Arborio rice
- 2 sprigs parsley, chopped (about 1 tablespoon)
- 1 celery stalk, chopped
- 1 medium onion, chopped
- 1 tablespoon olive oil

Method:

1. Press the sauté function of your instant pot. Add in the oil and once it is hot, add the onion and sauté until it begins to soften.

2. Add in the parsley and celery and sauté for around a minute.

3. Add in the garlic cloves and rice. Mix well and sauté until it is pearly; this should take around 1 minutes.

4. Select high pressure and cook for 5 minutes. Once time is up, allow pressure release and serve immediately. Swirl with some olive oil.

Chapter 4: Mediterranean Instant Pot Dessert Recipes

Baked Apples

Serves: 6

Cook Time: 20 minutes

Ingredients:

- 6 apples
- 1 teaspoon cinnamon powder
- ½ cup (100g) raw demerara sugar
- 1 cup (250ml) red wine
- ¼ cup (30g) raisins

Method:

1. Add the apples into the instant pot. Pour in the wine and add in cinnamon powder, sugar, and raisins. Close and lock the lid in place.

2. Cook at high pressure for 10 minutes. When the time is up, allow natural pressure release (around 20 minutes)

3. Serve the apples with some cream.

Peanut Butter Chocolate Cheesecake

Serves: 12

Ingredients:

- 3 eggs
- 24 ounces cream cheese
- 1 ½ tablespoons cocoa
- 3 tablespoons powdered peanut butter
- ¾ cup swerve sugar substitute
- 1 ½ teaspoons vanilla extract
- Whipped cream and peanut butter to top

To serve:

- Heavy cream
- Peanut butter, melted
- Roasted peanuts

Method:

1. Add all the ingredients into a blender and blend for 30-40 seconds or until smooth. Divide and pour into 12 mason jars. Cover the jars with lid or foil.

2. Pour 2 cups of water into the instant pot. Place a trivet in the pot.

3. Place as many jars as possible on the trivet. Cook the remaining jars in batches.

4. Close the lid. Select 'Manual' button and timer for 15 minutes.

5. Chill overnight.

6. Drizzle some heavy cream and peanut butter on the chilled cheesecake. Sprinkle roasted peanuts on top and serve.

Pots de Crème au Citron

Serves: 9

Ingredients:

- 9 egg yolks
- 1 ½ cups whole milk
- 1 cup sugar
- 1 ½ cups fresh cream
- 1 large lemon
- ¾ cup blackberries to garnish
- Blackberry syrup to top

Method:

1. Peel the lemon using a potato peeler. Use the peels in the recipe.

2. Add milk, lemon peels and cream into a heavy bottomed saucepan and place it over medium heat. Remove from heat when it just begins to bubble. Let it cool.

3. Whisk together yolks and sugar until sugar dissolves completely. Pour the cooled milk mixture into this and whisk until well combined.

4. Divide and pour into 9 ramekins and cover each ramekin with foil.

5. Pour 1 ½ cups water into the instant pot. Place a steamer basket in it.

6. Place the ramekins over it. Cook in batches if they all do not fit.

7. Close lid. Select 'Manual' button and timer for 10 minutes.

8. Let pressure release naturally. Remove ramekins. Uncover and set aside to cool. Place in the refrigerator until chill.

9. Garnish blackberries and drizzle blackberry syrup over it and serve.

Flan de Queso

Serves: 6

Ingredients:

- ¼ cup sugar
- 4 ounces reduced-fat cream cheese, (Neufchatel), softened
- 7 ounces canned nonfat or low-fat sweetened condensed milk
- 1 teaspoon vanilla extract
- 1 tablespoon water
- 4 large eggs
- ½ a 12-ounce can nonfat or low-fat evaporated milk

Method:

1. Add sugar and water into a small saucepan. Place over medium heat. Swirl the pan until the solution turns golden brown. Do not stir.

2. Pour immediately into a metal cake dish. Swirl the pan immediately so that the caramel spreads all over the bottom of the pan. Set aside. It will harden in a while.

3. Meanwhile, beat cream cheese with a stick blender or mixer on medium speed until soft.

4. Add an egg at a time. Beat well each time. Add condensed milk, evaporated milk, and vanilla extract. Stir until well combined.

5. Pour the mixture into the prepared pan.

6. Place a trivet inside the instant pot. Pour 2 cups of water.

7. Place dish over the trivet.

8. Close the lid. Select 'Manual' button and timer for 25 minutes. Let steam the release naturally. Cool completely.

9. Cover and refrigerator for 5-6 hours.

10. Run a knife all around the edges of the pan and invert on to a plate and serve.

Pears Stewed in Red Wine

Serves: 4

Cook Time : 5 to 10 minutes

Ingredients:

- 4 tablespoons heavy cream, dairy free
- 1 cup frozen raspberries
- 3/4 cup red wine
- 4 firm pears, peeled with stems on
- 1/4 teaspoon mace
- 2 cinnamon sticks
- 2 slices lemon
- 1/2 cup sugar
- 2 cups water

Method:

1. Mix together mace, cinnamon sticks, lemon, sugar and water in an Instant Pot. Simmer to dissolve the sugar.

2. Into the steamer basket, add the pears then lower into Instant Pot. Lock the lid and cook for 2 minutes at high pressure.

3. Quick release pressure and open the lid. Now add in red wine.

4. Lock the lid and cook for another 2 minutes then quick release pressure. Lift out the steamer basket and move the pears into a deep container.

5. Simmer the sauce on sauté function until syrupy. Pour over the pears.

6. To serve, puree raspberries in a blender, and then spoon 4 tablespoons of the puree on serving bowls.

7. Put a pear in each dish, then spoon over the sauce and raspberries then put a dollop of cream over the sauce.

8. Swirl the cream into the sauce using a knife to make a creative design.

I Need Your Help...

I want to thank you once again for choosing this book and hope you have had a good time cooking these dishes for your loved ones.

The Mediterranean diet is not a fad diet; it is a lifestyle diet that will provide you long-term results and lasting changes in your health. This book consists of recipes from different corners of the Mediterranean zone. All the recipes mentioned in this book are easy to cook, with simple, everyday ingredients.

It is all about getting started and bringing about lasting changes in your lifestyle. So what are you waiting for? Let's get started!

Finally, if you enjoyed this book, then I'd like to ask you for a favor, would you be kind enough to leave a review for this book on Amazon? It'd be greatly appreciated!

I want to reach as many people as I can with this book, and more reviews will help me accomplish that!

If you have any questions or problems, please contact us: hello@freedomdestination.com

Thank you and good luck!

Preview of 'Air Fryer Cookbook'

Firstly, you need to appreciate that despite the name, no frying happens in this appliance. Since the common understanding of frying usually means to cook in fat, the air fryer does not do that.

The Air fryer is a countertop convection oven (meaning it is an oven with a fan inside) that is self-contained and has a vertical orientation—the fan located at the top blows down through an electric heating component. The airflow begins at the top, heats up, and then moves fast around your food through a netting-cooking basket, and then down to a shaped drip tray that circulates the air back to the top. To use the device, you position the food you intend to 'fry' at the center of this airflow.

The mesh basket, so you know, resembles a deep fry basket. In this appliance, you will not find an oil reservoir or anything like it.

The General Features and Benefits of the Air Fryer

The air fryer has the following features and benefits:

Promotes low fat

First, you don't even have to add any oil when you are air-frying frozen food that is meant to be used for baking. You only need to take the food from the freezer, place it directly into the air fryer, and then set the temperature and timer. For raw meat, you also do not require any oil; the quick circulating hot air will cook your meat at all angles to give your meat a crispy outside and a moist inside. The excess fat from the meat will drip down the tray right below the cooking basket.

With the air fryer, you can try fried chicken wings, meat patties, pork chops, hot air dried fish, roast chicken, crackling roast pork, steaks and all other meat dishes you love.

It's automatic

While using the air fryer, the cooking process is a simple one. We have two popular types of hot fryers on retail: the paddle Tefal Actifry, and the mesh bottom-cooking basket that sits on a drip tray.

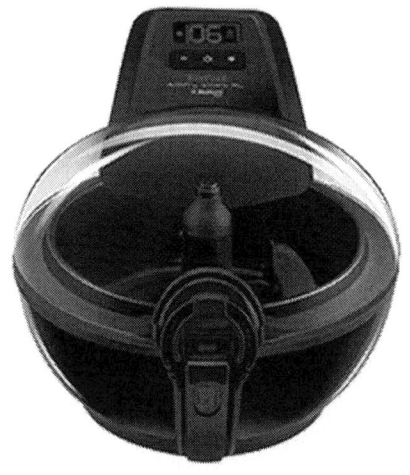

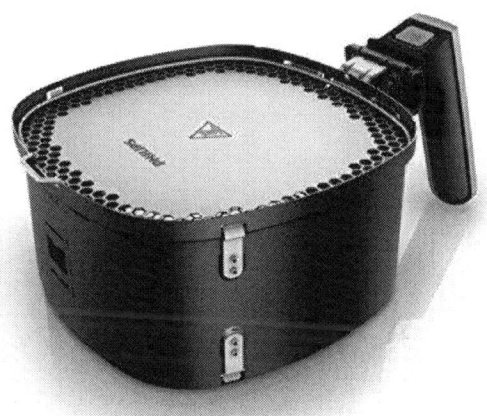

The former is the only one that comes with a stirring paddle; the other hot fryer brands in the market use the cooking basket design. You may also have noted that these hot fryers usually have their own air fryer accessories.

When using the Tefal Actifry air fryer, the only thing you have to do is place the chopped ingredients inside the cooking bowl. The machine will do the entire cooking process for you; the stirring paddle stirs the food gently as the bowl rotates. This definitely frees up your time for other things like making some salad to go with your food. Otherwise, you can just sit there and wait for the timer to beep when the food is ready.

NOTE: For the basket-style air fryer, you may need to shake the tinier cuts or flip the larger cuts over halfway through the cooking.

This machine is therefore incomparable with the hob cooking or the traditional stove that forces you to stand in front of the hot stove for the entire cooking process.

Imagine you are rushing to work in the morning; the last thing you want is to start cleaning up the usual mess after preparing breakfast. The hands-free and quick cooking quality the air fryer brings makes it win over the frying pan or skillet.

It's fuss-free

The air fryer only has 2 buttons, thus making it easy to use the air fryer. By adjusting the temperature and the timer, the meal will be ready when the timer goes off.

The Tefal Actifry makes things even easier because it only has the timer: the temperature setting is fixed. While hot air cookers usually come with pre-set programs, if you are unsure of the right temperature or cooking time, you can press the button for the type of food you are cooking. For instance, if you are cooking chicken, you just press the chicken icon button. The shortcut starter buttons takes out the guesswork out of air frying: fuss-free and simple!

Quick and convenient

You do not need to preheat the compact air fryer before you start cooking. You can easily transfer your frozen French Fries, nuggets, potato wedges and other ingredients directly into the fryer. Adjust the timer and temperature and a few minutes later, beep! Your food is ready.

Perhaps you feel like eating some roasted walnuts or groundnuts while watching football. That is no longer a big deal. Just wash them, place them in the air fryer, and wait to hear the beep.

Additionally, crispy food remains crispy when you reheat it. I do not know about you but I think this is better than buying fat and salt laden food at the fast food joints.

Finally, when cooking smaller food portions, you will find this gadget more practical than the ordinary convection oven. The fryer cooks faster and is economical too (concerning time and fuel consumption).

It's a multi-cooker

A machine that bakes, fries, grills, and roasts is undeniably a highly versatile appliance. Think about it; you have a deep fryer, toaster, skillet, hot grill, and an oven all fitted into one machine! You can use the air fryer for lunch, breakfast, and dinner to make sandwiches, grilled pork chop for dinner, and even snacks for lunch.

As you already know, we are living in a fast-paced world. The extremely versatile hot air fryer brings simplicity, ease, convenience, and so much more to your cooking process; if you do not like cooking, the air fryer's inventor must have had you in mind when inventing the device!

It's easy to clean

The best part is that all the air cooker's removable parts are dishwasher-safe. If you do not own a dishwasher, just soaking and gentle rubbing the parts with a clean sponge is good enough to get rid of all the bits of food stuck on the cooking surface.

Moreover, the appliance comes with a cover and you do all the cooking inside the machine. Unlike the oven or deep fryer, skillet or frying pan that all have an exposed cooking surface, with the air fryer, you will not find oil vapors deposited on your counter top, floor, or walls. This means the only thing that requires cleaning is the drip pan and cooking basket.

It is a food separator and food filter

Some cool air fryers available in the market today have a food separator that lets you cook multiple foods at the same time. For instance, if you want to prepare frozen chicken nuggets and French fries, you can use a separator to prepare the two simultaneously and while doing so, keep the flavors from mixing.

The air fryers also come with an air filter that ensures all the unwanted food odors and vapors do not spread around the house. Once you start using this device, you will have no more wafting food smells coming from your house since the air filter diffuses the hot air steam that floats and sticks. You will thus be able to enjoy your fresh kitchen smell before you start cooking, when you are cooking, and even after cooking.

So how exactly can an air fryer help you to become healthier? That's what we will discuss next.

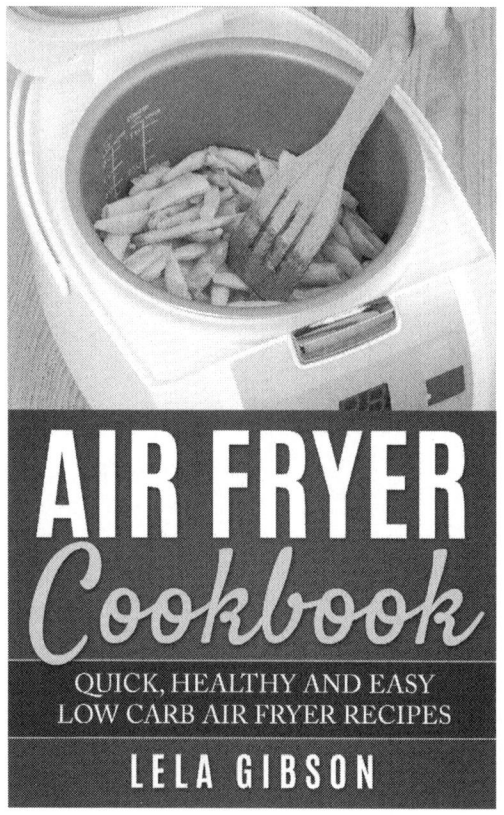

Check out the rest of Air Fryer Cookbook: Quick, Healthy and Easy Low Carb Air Fryer Recipes on Amazon, go to: http://amzn.to/2icNEqE

Check Out My Other Books

Below you'll find some of my other popular books that are popular on Amazon and Kindle as well.

Alternatively, you can visit my author page on Amazon to see other work done by me.

Instant Pot: Instant Pot Pressure Cooker Cookbook With Easy And Healthy Recipes

Dash Diet: Cookbook for Weight Loss with Action Plan and Easy Recipes

Slow Cooker: Cookbook With Slow Cooker Recipes

Anti-Inflammatory Diet Guide: The Guide to Reduce Inflammation and Live A Healthy Life Without Pain

Negative Calorie Diet: Cookbook & Guide Which Will Help You to Burn Body Fat, Lose Weight and Live Healthy

Anti-Inflammatory Diet Guide: The Guide to Reduce Inflammation and Live a Healthy Life Without Pain

Negative Calorie Diet & Dash Diet Box Set

Negative Calorie Diet & Weight Loss Box Set

Intermittent Fasting: The Essential Beginners Guide for Women for Weight Loss

Negative Calorie Diet & Anti-Inflammatory Diet Guide Box Set

Slow Cooker & Instant Pot Box Set

Negative Calorie Diet & Clean Eating Box Set

Leptin Resistance: Leptin Diet to Control Your Hormones, Get Permanent Weight Loss, Cure Obesity and Live Healthy

Weight Loss: 20 Easy and Fast Diet Tips for Losing Weight – an Easy-to-Follow Weight Loss Guide

Belly Diet: The Zero Belly Diet Step-by-Step Guide Which Helps You To Lose Your Belly and Enjoy Your Flat Belly

Belly Diet Smoothies: Delicious Smoothie Recipes to Flatten Your Belly, Improve Your Gut & Burn Fat

Weight Loss Cookbook: Meal Prep Cookbook For Weight Loss and Clean Eating

Smart Fat: Cookbook with Fat Meals Which Help You to Lose Weight, Get Healthy and Improve Brain Function

Clean Eating: Cookbook and Guide to Restore Your Body's Natural Balance and Eat Healthy

Negative Calorie Diet & Smart Fat Box Set

Weight Loss: 20 Easy and Fast Diet Tips for Losing Weight – an Easy-to-Follow Weight Loss Guide

Paleo Smoothies: Recipes to Energize and for Ultimate Health and Weight Loss

Ketogenic Cookbook: Quick Low Calorie Ketogenic Crockpot Recipes with 7 Days Meal Plan

Air Fryer Cookbook: Quick, Healthy and Easy Low Carb Air Fryer Recipes

Bonus: Subscribe To The Free Weight Loss Report

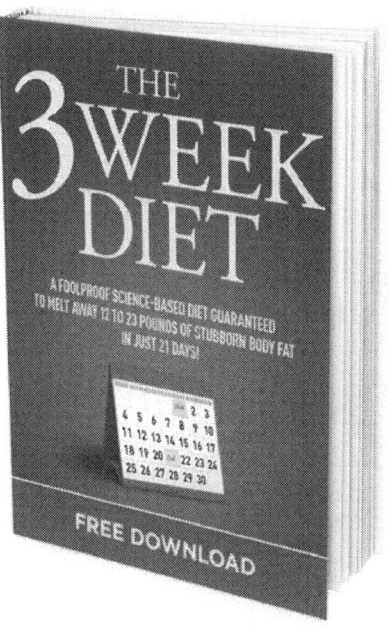

When you subscribe to https://freedomdestination.com/the-3-week-diet/ via email, you will get free access to an ebook. All you have to do is enter your email address to get instant access.

The Introduction Manual is more than just an introduction to the diet. Instead, it discusses the science behind how we gain and lose weight as well as what absolutely needs to be done to attack that stubborn body fat that, until now, has been so challenging to get rid of.

Here are the preview of what you'll get:

- Rapid Weight Loss
- How This System Works
- Why This Diet
- Why 3 Weeks?
- 21 Days To Make A Habit
- Fat Loss VS. Weight Loss
- Nutrients
- Protein, Fat, Carbohydrates
- The Food Pyramid And Obesity
- Fiber
- Metabolism
- How We Get Fat
- Triglycerides
- How To Get Thin
- Diet Overview
- Meal Frequency
- Water
- Diet Essentials
- Let's Get Started

Printed in Great Britain
by Amazon